Living Comfortably with Fibromyalgia

JANET MOORE

Living Comfortably with Fibromyalgia

ISBN: 978-1-965642-16-0

DEDICATION

To my husband, Greg, who has walked with me for the last 20 years.
I appreciate your willingness to stand back and hold space for my healing and growth, to support my desire to help and encourage others
even after I retired from my full-time nursing position.
To Mr. Ed, Ron Gainer, now deceased, who steadied me on my recovery journey. A true Christian Counselor who showed me what the love of Jesus looks like and helped so many people face their traumas
and heal together in community.
And to my Primary Care Physician, Michelle Tomczak, D.O., who, for more than 30 years, walked this dreadful journey with me through all the ups and downs, all the health challenges and mental health issues. I am forever grateful to have a physician who supported me on my journey and never made me feel like I was making things up or a hypochondriac.
To every fibromyalgia patient who will pick up this book and browse through its chapters, I pray that you find something that inspires hope for your journey and provides tools to help you measure success.

Living Comfortably with Fibromyalgia

CONTENTS

.

INTRODUCTION

Shortly after retiring from nursing, I was driving to a physician appointment when I felt a distinct prompt: *Use your life experiences and fibromyalgia diagnosis to help other women. Write a book about your journey. It will help others who are suffering.*

At my appointment, my physician asked about my retirement plans. I told her, "I'm writing a book about my fibromyalgia journey." Pain, medications, diagnosis, hospitalization, alternative treatments, and the tools I used to reclaim my life are all parts of my story.

I was diagnosed more than thirty years ago. With the support of my Primary Care physician, I took control of my life, learned to live comfortably with fibromyalgia, and work full-time, more than 40 hours per week, in a hospital setting.

It was not an easy journey. Finding a way to live somewhat comfortably took about three years of introspection, journaling, counseling, and emotional support. It was a lot of trial and error, which I prefer to reframe as "test for success". It was hard work to face the reality of my situation and make different choices. I could have given in to prescription medications, muscle relaxants, and antidepressants. And I did it for a while.

I could have become physically disabled and applied for disability benefits. But that was not the life I wanted to live.

I had grown up caring for my mother, who suffered from chronic back pain due to a work-related injury. I knew I didn't want to follow that path. Instead, I pursued a career as a nurse, determined to care for others and ultimately, myself.

Now, I can share my journey and the steps I took to reclaim my health and well-being. There were losses, grieving, and emotional pain. There was also abuse and neglect. But three grandmothers loved me. Women I looked up to who taught me strength, perseverance, and how to trust God with any situation.

Using my nursing knowledge and life experiences, I transformed myself from someone broken and in severe pain to someone who took control of my situation and created a life worth living.

1 DIAGNOSIS AND DECISION-MAKING

I realize that saying, "living comfortably with fibromyalgia," is controversial. With over 30 years of experience, I feel compelled to share my journey.

Many people I meet cannot believe that I have fibromyalgia, as I do not constantly complain about pain, I am very active, and I worked full-time as a hospital nurse until I retired.

I take no prescription medicines to manage it. I decided to find an alternative approach. As a nurse, I understand the expected effects, side effects, and long-term consequences of medications. I have seen the consequences firsthand in many of my patients with chronic illness and in my mother, who suffered from chronic back pain for decades. I knew I did not want that life.

Receiving a diagnosis for a chronic, debilitating disease that causes widespread pain, has no cure, and no standard treatment can feel like a death sentence.

Fibromyalgia is a neuromusculoskeletal disorder causing pain, muscle spasms, sleep disturbances, brain fog, headaches, impaired flexibility, impaired mobility, and fatigue, to name just a few of the life-altering symptoms.

My primary care physician (PCP) had been treating widespread pain in my body and other common symptoms. My symptoms were more right-sided, which correlated with a farming accident in my teens. Right shoulder and right hip pain with muscle spasms and knots under my shoulder blade that plagued me daily.

Additionally, I had been involved in three automobile accidents within a short period. A front-end collision with a deer, a nasty rear-end collision that totaled the car and left me with severe upper back and neck pain, numbness and tingling down my arms, and unrelenting migraines. The third accident was another front-end collision.

My chest hit the steering wheel, causing blunt chest trauma. A few hospitalizations eventually led to my having to quit my job as a hospital nurse to take care of myself.

The worst pain I ever experienced was a searing pain across my upper back that felt like someone was tearing my skin and muscles apart. I screamed with each new sensation.

Thankfully, I had a compassionate nurse who listened to my complaints, did a thorough assessment, and informed me that I was experiencing severe muscle spasms. She reassured me that there was treatment and that I would find relief.

When I was diagnosed by a physiatrist (physician specializing in physical rehabilitation medicine) in the late 1990s, fibromyalgia was a vague, catch-all term for a group of symptoms with no readily identifiable cause. Trigger point assessment and medical history were the primary tools. It was almost a joke to be tagged with fibromyalgia by a medical professional. Women were diagnosed more often than men.

The only treatments were symptom management with prescription pain medications, muscle relaxants, and antidepressants.

In most cases, the patients leave feeling like they have lost their minds, and no one believes in their suffering.

The physiatrist explained that fibromyalgia was a chronic, progressive, debilitating disease characterized by fatigue and widespread pain. She didn't elaborate further as we had already discussed the myriad symptoms I had been dealing with.

The only treatments were symptom management with prescription medications, though some patients found some relief with physical therapy and massage therapy. The thought of someone intentionally rubbing my skin and muscles to relieve pain was absurd.
Didn't she know how much pain I was having?

She told me there was no cure. I would have to figure out how to live with fibromyalgia and all that it brings along with it. Lifestyle management and medications were in my future.

And so, my fibromyalgia journey began.

I returned to my PCP with the information, which just confirmed her thoughts as she had been treating me for a couple of years, symptomatically.

I told her I would take some over-the-counter pain medications to be able to continue working to help support my family. I had worked long and hard to become a nurse and did not want to give up my passion for helping others.

I also explained that I wasn't going to take this diagnosis lying down. I was going to fight to find an appropriate treatment program for myself so I could live a whole life, not controlled by pain and muscle spasms.

2 LIFE TAKES OVER

As both a nurse and a young mother, I felt it was my responsibility to care for others first, even disregarding my health. Taking care of my children, my husband, my mother, and my grandmother seemed more important to me than addressing my growing symptoms. I learned to push through the pain, ignoring my body's signals.

I continued working full-time at the hospital while managing my household. Over time, I began asking my physician for medications to deal with the pain, muscle spasms, sleepless nights, anxiety, and depression. Soon, I was on a regimen (of prescription medication) for high cholesterol, high blood pressure, and eventually diabetes. These conditions ran in my family but were exacerbated by stress and poor self-care.

My physician asked me, "What is your long-term plan?"

We had already discussed that fibromyalgia was a progressive, chronic condition.

My only response was, "Just get me through this next year."

Year after year, I continued to push through. Eventually, my body had had enough. I developed heart problems, which forced me to quit my hospital job.

Being home was both a relief and a burden. It was nice to be home with my boys. However, the financial stress of not working weighed on me, and the pain and fatigue became unbearable.

At this point, my husband and I made a difficult decision. Since we could no longer afford our house, we sold it and moved to an apartment owned by his parents. I worried about privacy and feeling obligated to them, but financially, it was necessary.

One day, a friend from our church asked if I was interested in working part-time at his flower shop. A few days a week, a few hours a day. It provided both income and a creative outlet.

Surprisingly, this minor adjustment improved my mental and emotional well-being. My children noticed the difference immediately. The boys enjoyed the changes in me. I was a little lighter emotionally despite the pain. They would giggle when I came home from work.

"Mom, we know where you've been," they would say. "You smell like flowers."

This simple, unrelated job helped me reconnect with joy. My physician and I began tapering some of my medications. Though I was still in pain, I felt a renewed sense of purpose and hope.

3 PIVOT

A few years later, I returned to nursing in a physician's office within walking distance of our home.

When I was hired, I was introduced to the entire office staff. It was an interdisciplinary addiction medicine practice featuring an Internal Medicine physician, a psychotherapist with an addiction counseling background, a massage therapist, an acupuncturist, a chiropractor, and ancillary staff who also taught yoga and tai chi. The office staff included an office manager, the physician's wife, a billing clerk, and a receptionist. The medical practice was bustling with activity. Confidentiality was of the highest regard.

The counselor offered to be a listening ear if I ever needed one. I believe he recognized my situation before I was ready to acknowledge it.

Moving into the rental was a mixed blessing. While my husband could afford the rent, he remained frugal with other household expenses. I continued to cover the costs of our children's needs, stretching my limited income. While his parents were not as intrusive as I had feared, the new arrangement came with its own set of obligations: hosting family gatherings, Sunday meals, and maintaining an image of family unity.

I was still battling pain and muscle spasms, yet I had not fully explored alternative treatments beyond medication. My new work environment at the physician's office reawakened my passion for medicine and patient care.

I began reading about addiction, gastrointestinal disorders, and other chronic illnesses, hoping to expand my knowledge to better support our patients. Many of them faced stigma, particularly those struggling with addiction. I felt a deep sense of purpose in helping them.

My growing interest in these topics created tension at home. One day, my husband invited our pastor over for an unannounced visit.

Confused, I asked the pastor why he was there. He gently explained that my husband was uncomfortable with the reading materials I brought home. Surprised, I pressed further. My husband admitted that my shifted focus on addiction literature triggered his memories of his younger brother's struggles with alcoholism.

This revelation led to a long overdue conversation about his past, his fears, and our marriage dynamics.

This moment marked a turning point. I realized that while taking steps to reclaim my professional identity, I also needed to address emotional and relational challenges at home. My healing journey was not just physical. It was also mental, emotional, and spiritual.

During this time, my adoptive father became ill, was diagnosed with terminal lung cancer, and passed away. He had been a lifesaver. My younger sister and I believe we had a past life connection to him. He taught me about blueprints, as I am a visual learner. And I learned the meaning of true love.

I was so overcome by family responsibilities, living in the apartment, I did not allow myself to grieve this loss.

P.S. This marriage ended in divorce. I had to take time to accept responsibility and decide to take steps to take care of myself. Leading up to the divorce, I did the emotional work and grieving that was a necessary part of my healing journey. The grief list was long!

Happy News! After I did all the hard work, I was given a precious gift: a new husband who created a safe space for my continued healing and personal growth.

4 DOWN A DARK HALLWAY

One day, after preparing a patient for their appointment, I overheard a comment. "Look, the nurse is high."
The words stung. I was only taking a mild prescription pain medication and muscle relaxant to manage my fibromyalgia. The implication made me question whether I was presenting myself as the competent nurse I aimed to be.

Seeking clarity, I scheduled an appointment with the addiction counselor. I had seen his clients enter his office downcast and defeated, but depart in an uplifted, brighter mood. He and I light-heartedly joked that if I entered his office, I might not come back out.

I frequently gazed in as I passed by. The room was long and dimly lit by a table lamp. Soft music playing in the background made it a comforting space. The sign on the door had been altered from "M. Ed" to "Mr. Ed" by his clients, referring to Mr. Ed, the talking horse from 1960s television shows. His clients left in an uplifted demeanor, regardless of how they entered.

The day I was scheduled to see him was like any other day of the week. That would soon change. As I entered the room, I remember thinking that I was walking into a dark hole and would probably be swallowed up by the universe. Instead, I was overwhelmed by love and warmth. I crumbled to the floor, unable to take a step closer to sit on the chair across the room.

He asked if I was okay.

"I'm okay. I am overwhelmed by the warmth and loving presence I am experiencing."

He reminded me that this was a safe space.

He handed me a box of tissues and asked if I needed help getting up off the floor. I declined. The place I was sitting was the most comfortable spot I had been in, as far as I could remember.

I breathed a deep sigh of relief.

I explained my reason for being there, the comment from the patient, and their support person about being high. I shared that I had fibromyalgia and had been treated with prescription pain medications, but desired to find an alternative. I was fully aware of the consequences of the path I was on.

He reminded me that our practice did what I was looking for: help people make different choices for their health and well-being.

We discussed my concerns about being the right person to care for and support our patients. He affirmed my place in this office setting.

"You are just the person to be working here, as the office nurse. And even more so now that you are recognizing your own needs and asking for help."

"We can meet at a time that suits your work schedule to support your desire to help yourself. Being aware is the first step. Acknowledging you need help is the second. Asking and seeking help is the third."

"You are well on your way to a healthier life."

He continued, "I will work with you to walk your decided road to healing and recovery. You are in control of your life and your future."

I bawled like a baby. It only takes one person who acknowledges your pain and situation and extends a hand of support to be one of the best gifts I've received.

My journey down the dark hallway was about to begin. I would have to face my reality. Reclaiming my life was the pathway. Warmth and light were becoming visible.

5 SURRENDER

"The only way out is through."

Those were hard words to hear. I had already endured so much difficulty; could I continue to persevere to the end? Yes. I decided to surrender to the process.

I could no longer push forward without addressing the reality of my situation.

I wanted to speed up my healing and recovery. I desired to get back to living a whole, fun, happy, pain-free, medication-free life. I had no idea how sick I was.

I was living outside of my body due to the pain. I was disconnected. The counselor was having trouble getting me to connect my external reality with my internal self. A group activity tracing an outline of our body on a sheet of freezer paper and coloring it in showed me how I was seeing myself. Black and Blue with only a glimmer of warmth near my heart. Eye-opening. And a turning point in my reconnection to myself.

He suggested a Gratitude Journal to shift my thoughts from negative and defeated to positive and hopeful. I was reluctant to do this. What is there to be thankful for when you are miserable?

Well, it is a proven fact that what you focus on magnifies or expands. Suppose I concentrate on the pain, more pain. If I focus on the hugs from my children, I find joy and receive more hugs! If I focus on what I'm thankful for, I see more things to be grateful for. I challenge you to try it.

In a second journal, I freely wrote to get a grasp on the pain and my feelings about it. I was also struggling in my marital relationship and had been seeing a counselor with my husband to resolve our issues.

One day, unexpectedly, my husband asked me about something I had written in my pain and feelings journal. I felt something inside me.

Hurt, anger, disappointment. I felt violated and betrayed. He had been reading my journal.

I shared this with the counselor, who affirmed my feelings as accurate and appropriate.

"Now, the healing journey can begin. You are finally connecting the dots."

6 BREATHE. DECIDE. FIGHT.

After years of pushing through the pain, I reached a point where I had to make a choice: either continue down the same path of suffering and medication dependence or take control of my health in a new way. In my case, that meant Surrender.

I decided to fight for my new life.

But first, I had to take a breath.

Breathing became an essential part of my healing journey. I had spent years holding my breath literally and figuratively.

Stress, trauma, and chronic pain had conditioned me to take shallow, restricted breaths. I didn't realize how much this contributed to my fatigue and muscle tension. Through mindful breathing exercises, I began to reconnect with my body and create space for healing.

With a clearer mind, I started making deliberate choices to improve my quality of life. I adjusted my diet, focusing on anti-inflammatory foods. I committed to daily movement, even when my body protested.

I began to explore alternative therapies, including massage, acupuncture, and guided meditation. I added more intentional, focused prayer.

It wasn't easy. There were setbacks, moments of doubt, and days when the pain felt overwhelming. I reminded myself that this was a fight worth engaging in. I refused to let fibromyalgia define my existence.

Each day became an opportunity to reclaim a piece of myself. I journaled my progress, celebrating small victories. (I hid my journal from my husband.) I leaned on my support system- friends, family, and fellow fibromyalgia warriors. Slowly, I started to feel stronger, more in control, and hopeful for the future.

Choosing to fight did not mean that fibromyalgia disappeared. The pain was still there, but my relationship with it changed. I no longer viewed myself as a victim of my condition. Instead, I saw myself as an active participant in my healing.

This chapter of my journey speaks about the opportunity for a mindset shift and transformation. Breathing, deciding, and fighting became my first tangible steps toward living, not just surviving with fibromyalgia.

7 BUILDING MY "TOOLKIT"

Healing from fibromyalgia requires more than just accepting my diagnosis. It required action. I dislike the trial-and-error approach. My first massage therapist suggested the phrase, "test for success". She made suggestions based on my current level of pain, muscle spasms, and related fibromyalgia issues. We "tested for success". If something worked, "Score!" If it didn't, we set it aside. Sometimes it is not the right time to try a new treatment or modality.

Back to the Gratitude Journal.

Over time, I developed a personalized toolkit to help manage my symptoms and improve my quality of life. This toolkit became essential in my journey toward living comfortably with fibromyalgia.

Breathing. When I feel anxious, fearful, or stressed, I tend to stop breathing or hold my breath. I learned that this is a fight/flight response. I asked my support system to remind me to breathe if they noticed I wasn't. I still have quiet time, focusing on slow, deep, easy breaths.

Movement and exercise. While intense workouts often worsened my symptoms, gentle movement was essential to keep my muscles from stiffening and spasming. Gentle movements, such as stretching, reaching upward to the sky, bending over, touching my toes, twisting gently side to side, side bends, and knee lifts, help warm my body for the day's activities. I prefer a slow walk outside in the daytime or evening. Light weights assisted with strengthening the upper body and helped to maintain muscle tone without causing strain. My younger sister commented on my newly acquired muscle definition. Taichi became part of my daily routine, helping with balance and joint mobility. I added a vibration plate/shaker to my routine a few times a week, as it does not require physical exertion.

Nutrition and hydration. Since our bodies are mainly composed of water, and most of us do not enjoy drinking it, this was a challenging undertaking. I remembered trips to friendly hotels that had chilled water in a pretty dispenser and decided to try it at home. I drink at least half of my body weight in water daily. I prefer it to be chilled, but room temperature is satisfactory. You need to drink it. At first, I added lemon or lime. Orange slices were the key for me. It was pleasing to the eye and tasted great! Cucumbers, mint, apples, and berries are also good additions. To add essential minerals, I use Celtic salt. Only a small amount, equivalent to a grain or two, is needed. The food I ate played a crucial role in managing inflammation, pain, and maintaining my energy levels. I focused on whole, unprocessed foods, rich in nutrients. I minimized sugar and refined carbohydrates, which often triggered symptoms. I reduced my intake of caffeine, sugar, and simple carbohydrates. Too much white bread makes my knees and hips hurt. An anti-inflammatory diet helped with some of my symptoms.

Sleep and Rest. These are two different things. Fibromyalgia often disrupts my sleep, leading to chronic fatigue. Improving my sleep hygiene became critical. I had to establish a sleep routine that accommodates my lifestyle and work schedule. A regular bedtime with a regular get-up time. A more fabulous room, dark with an overhead fan. I chose not to have a television in my room. I prefer natural fabrics, such as cotton or bamboo sheets, and blankets of various textures and weights. A weighted blanket can provide comfort and help alleviate restless legs; the weight varies, so try a few different ones to find the one that works best for you. An electric blanket was comforting on cold nights. A heating pad with automatic shut-off to prevent accidental burns. Reusable heated packs. And occasional ice packs. An eye mask. Earplugs. A sound machine or soft music. A warm bath with Epsom salts or a shower with lavender-scented body wash. A warm cup of chamomile tea is a soothing bedtime treat. Magnesium glycinate, taken 30 minutes to 1 hour before bedtime, helped to relax my muscles and improve my sleep quality. Melatonin did nothing for me. An infrared sauna was a welcome addition.

Resting. A mid-afternoon nap was my grandmother's way of disconnecting from the day's busyness to rest and recharge. I do that now, too. Find a comfortable, cozy spot and curl up or stretch out. Quiet atmosphere or soft music. Lay still and focus on your breath, so, your body can relax. My mind was non-stop most of the time. To-do lists, accusations, shaming, and belittling. That crazy voice in my head, that needed to shut up! I found clary sage essential oil that acts like a chalkboard eraser, quieting the noise in my brain. It may or may not help you, but I think essential oils and aromatherapy are worth trying.

Emotional and Mental Well-being. Fibromyalgia affects more than just the body. It impacts the mind and emotions. Learning to manage stress and emotional triggers was key to my healing. I practiced deep breathing exercises and meditation to calm my nervous system. I used prayer to stay connected to God and share my concerns, worries, and fears. Journaling allowed me to process emotions and track symptom patterns. I sought therapy to work through past traumas, which I learned had played a role in my chronic pain. I got a divorce. And I built a support network of friends, family, and fellow fibromyalgia warriors to help me feel less isolated.

Boundaries and Self-care. One of the most challenging but necessary changes I made was setting boundaries. I learned to say "no" without guilt when my body needed rest. Sometimes I had to say "no" to social events or commitments that would overextend me, such as overtime at the hospital and late evening events that would disrupt my sleep routine. It took longer for me not to need to have an explanation for "no" every time I said it. I prioritized self-care without feeling selfish, understanding that I couldn't pour from an empty cup. I prioritized relationships that were supportive and uplifting. I removed toxic people and stressful obligations from my life without guilt. And No Negative Self Talk!

Massage therapy. This was probably the most challenging tool to add to my toolkit. I had such bad pain and sensitivity to touch that even the thought of massage therapy upset me. The addiction counselor referred me to a massage therapist with experience in caring for fibromyalgia patients. She was patient, understanding, and skilled in her approach. I started with 10–to 15-minute sessions once a week, gradually increasing the length of time as my body could tolerate. I worked my way up to one hour weekly. It is so beneficial to keep my symptoms under control and manage pain issues when they arise. Healthy physical touch is lacking in patients with chronic pain, and good medical professionals will tell you it is necessary for mental health.

Supplements. I began using calcium, magnesium, and zinc supplements early in my healing journey. My first massage therapist recommended them due to muscle functioning, spasms, and pain. I take it three times a day and know when I miss a dose or switch to a different brand. I also take a vitamin B complex, vitamin B12 weekly or more often if I am fatigued, and vitamin D3 with K2.

Pain management. Fortunately, I have little to no pain. Only on rare occasions do I take over-the-counter acetaminophen or naproxen. I use Salon Pas patches for the topical relief of muscle aches or pain. A topical magnesium lotion can help alleviate tightness and cramping. Additionally, my massage therapist in Florida recommends bio-freeze, lidocaine lotion or patches, and a Thai green lotion. These are used rarely, but are part of my toolkit, should I need them. Moist heat and ice are also beneficial for strains or injuries.

A creative pursuit or hobby. We were created to be creative. Perhaps you enjoy reading or watching television programs. You may prefer to spend time in the kitchen, cooking, baking, or creating a new dish. Painting, knitting, crocheting, drawing, visiting with someone, going on an adventure. Building, gardening, and taking things apart to see how they work. Spending time with family members, friends, or pets. All these activities tell our brain that we are someone special, with interests and desires that drive us to be productive and happy.

Healing is not linear. It is a journey filled with twists, setbacks, and unexpected discoveries. My experience with fibromyalgia was no exception. Once I accepted my diagnosis and built my toolkit, I had to learn how to implement these strategies into my daily life.
At first, progress felt frustratingly slow. I wanted immediate results for the pain and muscle spasms. Fibromyalgia does not allow for quick fixes. Instead, I had to redefine success.

Getting through a day with less pain than before became a win.

Completing a simple yoga session, even if modified, was an achievement.

Saying "no" to an event that might overextend me or because I needed rest became an act of self-love, not a failure.

By focusing on small victories, I kept myself motivated and prevented myself from falling into despair.

This shift in mindset allowed me to embrace a new normal where I was no longer fighting against my condition but working with it to create a life I could enjoy.

The following page was intentionally left blank so you could begin Building your Toolkit.

8 NON-NEGOTIABLES

As I continued to refine my approach to living comfortably with fibromyalgia, I realized that some aspects of my daily life were essential for maintaining my well-being.

These non-negotiables became the foundation of my daily life. Without them, my symptoms worsened, and I felt out of control. By committing to these essential habits, I regained a sense of empowerment and stability in my fibromyalgia.

Let's revisit Chapter 7: "Building My Toolkit," as most of these items became my non-negotiables.

Rest and Sleep
Hydration, especially water.
Daily movement
Gratitude
Massage therapy. Budget breaker? Not for me!
Magnesium supplements
Healthy boundaries
Something to look forward to

When I let up on any of these things in my toolkit, I begin to experience muscle spasms, pain, anxiety, and overall uneasiness.

My co-workers and others I met could not understand how I could afford weekly massage therapy. I asked them how much money they spent on a weekend out, including drinks, dinner, and other activities. Do you quickly drop $100 or more? At the time I began, the rate for massage therapy was $50 per hour. It is now close to $100 per hour, or more.

How can I afford it? It is a genuine question, as we spend a significant amount of money trying to find ways to take care of ourselves. We may not think we have the resources to do it. Massage therapy costs continue to rise, and skilled therapists may seem out of financial reach. As I have found that massage therapy is an excellent way to manage my symptoms, I made it non-negotiable. It is a budget line that does not come off the books.

When I looked at the cost of prescription medications and the side effects versus massage therapy, the cost of massage therapy is far less, and it provides only positive effects for me. I reviewed my discretionary spending and found that money can be easily saved by limiting fast-food stops, daily high-priced coffee drinks, alcohol added to meals on weekends, and subscriptions I no longer use, among other areas.

When I decided to review my spending, I looked at how much better I felt when using massage therapy as part of my treatment plan versus not doing it. Annually, while still working, I received a wage adjustment in my nursing position, which became my massage money.

If you are looking for a reasonably priced massage therapist for fibromyalgia, consider checking your local chiropractor's office for referrals. They usually employ a therapist as an adjunctive treatment for their patients. You can schedule an appointment in conjunction with a chiropractic adjustment. Some of these may also be covered by insurance.

Health Savings Accounts and Flexible Medical Spending Accounts often cover the cost of massage therapy, provided that a prescription from your physician and documentation from the therapist's practice are submitted.

My other non-negotiables are primarily behavioral and lifestyle changes that do not require financial investment.

I encourage you to identify your non-negotiables. What daily practice helps you feel your best? What boundaries do you need to set?

These choices will become the pillars of your wellness journey.

9 ANNUAL AND QUARTERLY REVIEWS

Managing fibromyalgia is an ongoing process, requiring adjustments and regular self-reflection. I found that conducting personal health reviews on an annual and quarterly basis helped me stay on track and make necessary changes to improve my quality of life.

Prioritizing Rest and Sleep

Fibromyalgia and fatigue go hand in hand. I had to create a structured sleep routine to support my body's need for recovery.

- Establish consistent bedtime and wake-up time, even on the weekends.
- Avoid caffeine and heavy meals in the evening to improve sleep quality.
- Invest in a supportive mattress and pillows to decrease nighttime pain.
- Use relaxation techniques, such as deep breathing and guided meditation, before bed to calm the mind and quiet the body.

Daily Movement, No Exceptions

Movement is necessary to prevent stiffness and reduce pain, even on difficult days.

- On good days, I engage in yoga, Taichi, walking, or light strength training.
- On flare days, I opt for gentle stretching or an extra few minutes of deep breathing exercises.
- I incorporate movement throughout my day, avoiding prolonged sitting

Nutrition that Supports Healing

The foods I ate played a crucial role in managing inflammation and energy levels.

- Focus on whole, unprocessed fruits and vegetables, rich in nutrients and fiber. High-quality protein is essential.
- Minimize sugar and refined carbohydrates, which often trigger symptoms. Artificial sweeteners are a "no" for me.

- Stay hydrated by drinking plenty of water infused with lemon, lime, orange, cucumber, or mint.

Boundaries and Saying "No"

Learning to set boundaries was one of the most powerful tools for protecting my mental and emotional health.

- I said "No" to social events or commitments that would overextend me.
- I prioritized relationships that were supportive and uplifting.
- I removed toxic people and stressful obligations from my life without guilt.

Emotional and Mental Health Care

Managing fibromyalgia wasn't just about the physical aspect; my emotional reactions needed adjustment, too.

- No negative self-talk. Be Kind.
- Start a Gratitude Journal. Write down three things each day that you are thankful for or that bring you joy.
- Build a supportive community.

Celebrating Resilience

Fibromyalgia may have changed my life, but it did not take away my strength and resolve. Every day I chose to show up for myself was proof of my resilience. I was no longer just surviving; I was creating a life that honored my needs, limitations, and capabilities. The journey was not perfect, but it was mine. And, for the first time in years, I felt like I was truly living.

Once a month, I would write out "My Ideal Life". What did I want my life to look like? I included the following categories:

Physical Health
Finances
Relationships
Mental Health
Spiritual Health

Physical Activity
Pain management
Other symptom management
Weight
Exercise
Creative pursuits or How I spend my free time
Rest and sleep
Nutrition and hydration

I love doing this. Setting a target for my success.

At the end of each year, I take time to reflect on how I managed my fibromyalgia.
- What worked well for me.
- What challenges did I face, and how did I handle them?
- Did my symptoms improve, worsen, or stay the same?
- Are there new treatments, therapies, or lifestyle changes I want to explore?

Revisit non-negotiables.
- Make necessary adjustments.
- If something no longer serves me, I thank it for the time it helped, and I release it.
- If I discovered a new strategy that improved my quality of life, I committed to incorporating it into my routine.

Do it as often as you wish. Your brain and body will begin to thank you as you update your vision for a healthier future.

The following page was intentionally left blank so you could begin writing "My Ideal Life".

MY IDEAL LIFE   DATE:_____

10 THE GIFTS OF FIBROMYALGIA

Regardless of the path you choose to deal with your fibromyalgia, there are still gifts to be discovered. I can see myself as diseased and disabled, or I can see myself as blessed with an infirmity.

In addition to my identity, this also encompasses my emotional state, physical being, and spiritual self.

I can embrace and love myself for who I was created to be. I am unique and have something to offer to those around me. I am One of a Kind!

I can celebrate being alive.

I can enjoy creative pursuits. I ask myself, 'How do I want to spend my time and energy today?'

I am an optimistic person by nature. I decided to dig into this new life of Living Comfortably with Fibromyalgia and found 10 Gifts.

They are as follows:
1. Self-awareness, mindfulness, and presence
2. Increased experiential empathy and compassion for others
3. Resilience and strength
4. Prioritized self-care
5. Connection to others
6. Creativity and expression
7. Gratitude
8. Spiritual growth
9. Meeting interesting people: i.e., others with fibromyalgia, physicians, office staff, helpers, counselors, authors, and speakers
10. An acceptable excuse to get out of doing anything I don't want to do

Conclusion

Living with fibromyalgia has been one of the most challenging journeys of my life, but it has also been one of the most formative. Through "test for success", I have learned that managing a chronic illness is not about eliminating pain; it is about finding ways to live fully despite it.

With the support of a counselor, I was able to face my traumas, reconcile my feelings that had been stuffed down, forgive myself and others, and learn to love authentically.

Thank you for reading my story. May you find comfort, strength, and hope as you continue your journey.

AUTHOR BIO

JANET MOORE is a wife, mother, grandmother, nurse, aspiring coach, and first-time author. Diagnosed over 30 years ago, she refused to let her condition define her. Instead, she embarked on a journey to discover alternative treatments, lifestyle changes, and mindset shifts that would enable her to live a fulfilling life. Today, she shares her experiences of inspiring and supporting others who face similar challenges.
When she is not writing or speaking about fibromyalgia, she enjoys time with family and friends, cooking, baking, sewing, and crocheting. She serves in her local church and spends time connecting with others in the chronic illness community.

For more information related to Fibromyalgia, please visit www.fibromyalgiasupportnetwork.com. Janet has a private Facebook group called "Living Comfortably with Fibromyalgia."

www.ingramcontent.com/pod-product-compliance
Lightning Source LLC
Chambersburg PA
CBHW070218300326
41934CB00036BA/3225